REGULATING NERVOUS SYSTEM DYSREGULATION

A step-by-step guide to reverse Mental

Health and promote well-being

By Judy Strickland

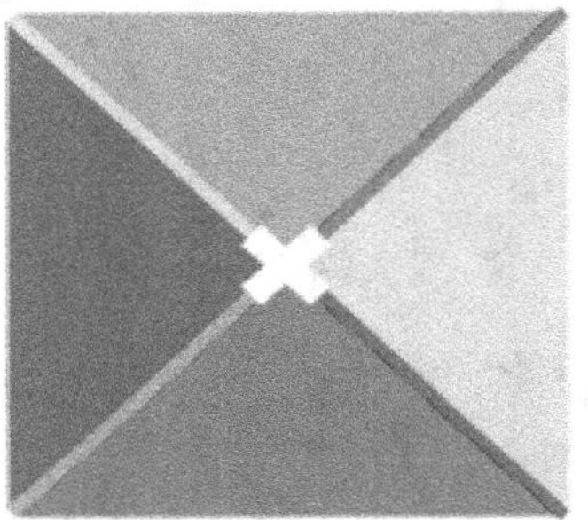

DISCLAIMER:

CHAPTER 1: Dysregulated Nervous System Definition

Introduction

One of the main indicators of psychological dysfunction in a variety of mental health disorders is nervous system dysregulation.

It can have a serious impact on our ability to make decisions, how we view the world, and how we interact with people regularly.

If the symptoms are severe enough and long enough, they can also impact our sense of self and make us feel powerless.

This explains why many healing processes depend so heavily on a neural system that is in balance.

Our experiences with the nervous system tell us if we are safe or not, which encourages more symptomatic reactions.

Regaining control over your neurological system is therefore essential to improving your quality of life.

The Nervous System: What Is It?

You can think of the nervous system as the body's control center.

All of these anatomical regions, as well as many more, are linked together by the neurological system. The heart, brain, and stomach all indeed have important roles to play in how you operate and interact with the outside world.

Your neurological system has an impact on every aspect of your health.

Anatomically, your nervous system is divided into two primary regions:

The brain and spinal cord make up the central nervous system (CNS) of your body. It aids in the regulation of bodily temperature, breathing, heart rate, movement, emotion, and cognition.

Outer Nervous System: The nerves that radiate from your central nervous system comprise your peripheral nervous system. Your limbs, glands, and organs are among the parts of your body that get messages from these nerves.

Additionally, the peripheral nervous system is composed of two components:

A large portion of your body's mobility is controlled by your somatic nervous system (SNS). It conveys messages from your brain to your body, so you may move it consciously and use your senses of taste, smell, hearing, and touch.

The body's involuntary physiological activities are regulated and controlled by the autonomic nervous system (ANS). The sympathetic, parasympathetic, and enteric nervous systems make up this system.

Nervous system dysregulation: what is it?

Chronic dysregulation of the neurological system might lead to a person's response to outside stimuli that isn't consistent with reality.

With time, this may result in a variety of physical, mental, and emotional health problems, as well as nerve dysregulation events.

However, several things, such as traumatic experiences, ongoing stress, or inherited tendencies, could cause this. Dysregulation of the nervous system prevents it from carrying out its functions effectively, leading to a host of symptoms, including chronic stress or worry, burnout, and a variety of chronic pain or illnesses.

Nervous system dysregulation can significantly impact the majority of bodily processes can be significantly impacted by nervous system dysregulation. Many people are unable to begin the transition to a more regulated state because they are unaware that this is the fundamental source of many of the symptoms they encounter.

Symptoms of a dysregulated nervous system

The initial step towards achieving optimal health and regulation is identifying the signs and manifestations of a dysregulated neural system. Here are some physical and psychological indicators of a dysregulated neural system are as follows:

1. **You feel stressed and tense all the time.**

   Feeling overwhelmed is one of the most obvious symptoms of nervous system dysfunction. Although it may seem illogical, this occurs when you find it difficult to let go of things or when you feel as though there are always too many demands on your time and attention.

   It's possible that you feel overwhelmed by everything and are constantly on edge, wondering what's going to happen next.

   Even when things appear to be going well, you frequently feel overwhelmed and stressed out.

   You find it hard to unwind. It's challenging for you to rest and quiet your mind sufficiently. You may find yourself constantly thinking or worrying about your relationships, future, and to-do list.

2. You tend to be impulsive, agitated, and sensitive.

Do you feel as though you're about to lose your temper or snap at any moment? This can indicate that you're having trouble controlling your emotional stress.

You can experience simultaneous agitation and frustration. An emotional reaction might be triggered by seemingly insignificant things because it feels like there's too much pressure building up within you.

It's like you tend to overreact in some circumstances. It gets harder for you to regulate your emotions or reactions. This could have an impact on your relationships and self-perception.

If your emotions are wildly fluctuating without any prior notice or building, you could be wondering why you are unable to regulate your responses and sentiments.

It's like you tend to overreact in some circumstances. It gets harder for you to regulate your emotions or reactions. You might get angry, impatient, and upset easily. Your mood abruptly swings from being depressed to being joyful for no apparent reason.

3. You experience chronic pain and illness.

Life stressors such as sickness, trauma, unfavorable childhood experiences, and persistent stress can lead to nervous system dysregulation. Over time, any kind of neural system dysfunction can lead to chronic pain and sickness.

Let's say that despite seeing numerous physicians, specialists, chiropractors, physical therapists, and others, you were only able to receive short-term alleviation and no lasting answers. This suggests that you may be suffering from nervous system dysregulation.

Additionally, you might have flare-ups and symptoms without a clear cause or trigger. This is frequently an indication that your body has been in a state of high sympathetic arousal for a considerable amount of time, which can cause a variety of physical issues over time.

Even if you try to eat healthily and exercise, you might have pain or illness for an extended period. It could seem as though your symptoms would never go away. It's not only physical; sometimes you have problems focusing on anything but how excruciating the ache in your head when you sleep is.

4. **You're highly sensitive to sensory stimuli.**

Strong sensory inputs quickly overwhelm you, and you most likely consider yourself to be a highly sensitive person (HSP). It can be difficult to control loud noises, specific smells, large crowds, particular noises, and other sensory inputs.

In addition, you react strongly to pain and become quickly upset or disturbed over seemingly insignificant things, such as clutter or the sound of gum being chewed. Your constant overload of sensory information may cause you to experience fear, anxiety, or depression.

A low threshold for sensory input is common in HSPs. You may find distractions from blazing lights, loud noises, and strong scents. These stimuli may even feel painful or unpleasant to you.

5. You have trouble falling asleep and are tired during the day.

You experience restless nights and fatigue during the day. During the day, you may find yourself yawning, drowsy, or sluggish and struggling to focus.

Dysregulation of the nervous system can disrupt sleep cycles. This is a result of your neurological system's inability to decompress when you sleep.

It's also possible that you have trouble controlling your heart rate and temperature, which makes it hard to fall asleep at night. Despite the room's temperature, you may experience a persistently higher heart rate or feel excessively hot or chilly. And because of these problems controlling your body's processes, you can be lying awake for the whole night.

You may lack the energy to enjoy activities with friends, family, or coworkers or to complete your regular responsibilities. You find it difficult to become motivated when you're constantly tired.

6. Chronic attention and concentration problems.

You find it difficult to concentrate on conversations or work. Because your nervous system is constantly scanning for danger, it is difficult to focus when it is fully alert.

Your body remains alert even when there is no threat, which makes it difficult to concentrate or focus on long-term objectives.

Perhaps you misplace items, neglect to turn in schoolwork, become distracted when conversing with others, or experience all of these symptoms at once! You believe that other individuals are more capable and intelligent than you are.

7. **Cravings and extreme appetite changes.**

There may be fluctuations in your appetite. One may have constant hunger or feel as though they are not eating enough. This is because your body's stress hormones are always fluctuating, which might alter how hungry you are.

Alternatively, it could simply be episodes of binge eating without a clear cause: you might be eating normally for a while, then all of a sudden feel the desire to eat a lot of sugar, salt, or fat.

If you find it difficult to control your eating habits, there may be a problem with the way your neurological system controls your body's metabolism.

8. **Immunity and hormonal symptoms.**

Since your neural system controls every bodily function, hormone abnormalities and a diminished or heightened immune response to stimuli are two of the most prevalent signs of dysregulation.

9. **Skin and Gut Conditions**.

Individuals with disorders such as IBS and Rosacea frequently experience dysregulation of their neurological systems. They frequently hear advice to "reduce stress" in their lives, but they struggle to know how to start and stop the healing process. Rosacea and IBS disappear when they take care of their nervous system's health and build a robust, balanced system.

10. **You're highly sensitive to other people's emotional states.**

One could define you as an empath. However, over time, your mental and physical health will be harmed by your oversensitivity to other people's emotional states. Even when someone doesn't ask for it, you feel compelled to look after them. You never seem to be able to do enough, and you eventually run out of energy. As a result, you become angry and bitter toward the person who stole your energy.

It's imperative to recognize these symptoms since unchecked dysregulation of the neurological system can result in severe symptoms. Chronic dysregulation over time may be linked to immune system weakness, sleep disorders, anxiety, burnout, and chronic pain issues.

What is the Impact of Nervous System Dysregulation on Your Mental Health?

The sympathetic and parasympathetic nervous systems are the main nervous system components that influence most mental health issues.

An important function is also played by the limbic system, which is a component of the central nervous system that is connected to the brain.

The Nervous-Sympathetic System

A portion of our survival mechanism is powered by the sympathetic nervous system.

Over millions of years, our sympathetic nervous system has developed to defend us against imagined dangers from predators, emotional strain, and other traumatic events.

The production of adrenaline, epimerase, and other stress-signaling chemicals, as well as an elevated heart rate, fast breathing, and muscle contraction, are all results of an active or triggered sympathetic nervous system.

Rather than accepting our fate inertly, these processes have developed to assist us in identifying and evading danger.

Living in cities now, we are not in nearly as much danger as our forefathers were.

Even so, the sympathetic nervous system—which is a component of the autonomic nervous system—remains an essential component of the human experience and operates autonomously.

That is to say, even in situations where there isn't a genuine threat, dysregulation can occur.

Sympathetic dominants are those who primarily experience dysregulation of the sympathetic nervous system.

Thus, when there is a risk or a perception of danger, the person will experience hyperarousal.

This is the classic fight-or-flight response.

The Nervous System of the Parasympathetic

Sometimes referred to as the "feed and breed" or "rest and digest" portion of the nervous system, the parasympathetic nervous system is situated between the brain and spinal cord.

The parasympathetic nervous system is needed to control the body's hyperactive processes once the sympathetic nervous system has taken hold.

Hence, to some extent, the parasympathetic nervous system helps to mitigate the consequences of the sympathetic nervous system.

It also helps with reproduction, digestion, and returning the body to a secure state.

In addition to affecting the heart and breathing rate and quality, the parasympathetic nervous system also releases stress chemicals like cortisol and others, which help the body return to a balanced condition.

However, the parasympathetic nervous system is also capable of inducing instability in itself.

The freeze and fawn phases of nervous system dysregulation, which can also result in dissociation, are under parasympathetic control.

It is said to be parasympathetic-dominating if they frequently enter frozen or fawning states.

Summing Up

Nervous system dysregulation is a significant indicator of psychological dysfunction in mental health disorders, impacting decision-making, worldview, and social interactions. It can lead to feelings of powerlessness and affect healing processes. The nervous system, which includes the heart, brain, and stomach, is the body's control center and plays a crucial role in various aspects of health.

The central nervous system (CNS) regulates bodily temperature, breathing, heart rate, movement, emotion, and cognition, while the peripheral nervous system (PNS) controls limbs, glands, and organs. The somatic nervous system

(SNS) controls mobility and the autonomic nervous system (ANS) regulates involuntary physiological activities. Chronic dysregulation can result in physical, mental, and emotional health problems, including chronic stress, burnout, and chronic pain or illnesses.

Symptoms of a dysregulated nervous system include feeling stressed and tense all the time, being impulsive, agitated, and sensitive, experiencing persistent discomfort and sickness, and receiving short-term relief from various treatments. Flare-ups and symptoms without a clear cause or trigger may indicate a prolonged state of high sympathetic arousal, leading to physical issues over time.

Regaining control over the neurological system is essential for improving quality of life and preventing symptoms. By identifying these indicators and manifestations, individuals can begin to transition to a more regulated state and improve their overall well-being.

Dysregulation of the nervous system can lead to various physical and mental health issues. It can cause a person to experience intense pain, difficulty falling asleep, fatigue, and difficulty concentrating on tasks. The nervous system's inability to decompress during sleep can disrupt sleep cycles and cause problems controlling heart rate and temperature, making it difficult to fall asleep at night.

Long-term difficulties with focus and attention may also occur due to the constant scanning for danger by the nervous system. Severe appetite fluctuations and cravings may also occur due to fluctuating stress hormones or episodes of binge eating. Immunity and hormonal symptoms are common signs of dysregulation, as the nervous system controls every bodily function.

Individuals with disorders such as IBS and Rosacea often experience dysregulation of their neurological systems. These disorders can be treated by addressing their nervous system's health and building a robust, balanced system.

The sympathetic and parasympathetic nervous systems are the main components that influence most mental health issues. The sympathetic nervous system is responsible for our survival mechanism, producing adrenaline, epimerase, and other stress-signaling chemicals, as well as an elevated heart rate, fast breathing, and muscle contraction. Sympathetic dominants experience hyperarousal when there is a risk or perception of danger.

The parasympathetic nervous system, situated between the brain and spinal cord, helps control the body's hyperactive processes and regulates reproduction, digestion, and returning the body to a secure state. It also releases stress chemicals like cortisol to help the body return to a balanced condition. However, it can also induce instability in itself, as seen in the freeze and fawn phases of nervous system dysregulation.

CHAPTER 2: Nervous System Dysregulation: Risk Factors and Causes

What are the causes of nervous system dysregulation?

The SNS and PNS are intended to function in unison, with collaboration and ease of use. The PNS has the potential to seriously damage the body if it malfunctions. When your body is out of balance and your sympathetic nervous system is activated more frequently than usual, it gradually deteriorates due to the system's loss of control.

A few of the contributing factors are enumerated below:

1. **Psychological Aspects: Trauma and Stress**

   Stress and trauma are the primary contributors to a dysregulated neurological system. Perceived stress affects many neuroendocrine systems through a process called experience-dependent plasticity. Stress causes dysregulation of the neurological system by upsetting the hormonal, autonomic, and subcortical systems, causing dysregulation of the neurological system.

   Trauma has an impact on homeostasis or self-regulation, the ability of biological systems to remain stable while adapting to a constantly changing environment. It is charged with preserving the organism's physiological equilibrium.

   Stress from trauma can make it harder to keep control over our emotions and experiences, which might throw off our nervous system. Someone who has a malfunctioning neurological system is unable to regain homeostasis.

2. **Lifestyle and Biochemical Elements**

Neurological dysregulation is also linked to lifestyle and biochemical factors. Biochemical factors include intestinal problems, toxicity, and infection. Difficult situations, such as financial hardship, bereavement, social troubles, and significant life events like the death of a loved one, divorce, or pregnancy, are examples of lifestyle and behavioral factors.

These substances trigger neuroendocrine chain reactions in the neuroendocrine system. Therefore, our bodies may perceive an ongoing assault by toxins like mold or heavy metals, infections like Lyme disease or Bartonella, or pathogens in our gut as a serious threat to our physiology.

Our bodies are made to defend against these kinds of attacks, so when we encounter one, our nervous system may go into overdrive and release stress hormones, which may, if unchecked, result in inflammation.

Identify the underlying causes and conditions that could lead to nervous system dysregulation.

Many things can lead to a neurological system that is dysregulated. The following are a few of the main reasons:

1. **Chronic stress:** is one of the most common causes of neural system dysregulation. Your neurological system is on high alert when your body is constantly under stress. An overreaction to stress might eventually lead to overwhelm and hypervigilance.

   Furthermore, how people view and manage their stress is a critical factor. Maladaptive attitudes or inadequate coping mechanisms, for example, can intensify the body's stress reaction.

2. **Stress:** Dysregulation of the neurological system can result from both physical and emotional stress. This covers things like mishaps, medical procedures, maltreatment, or being present at upsetting events.

3. **Adverse Childhood Experiences (ACEs):** Adverse childhood experiences can affect how the nervous system develops and lead to dysregulation. Examples of these events include physical or emotional abuse, neglect, and living with a family member who struggles with mental illness or substance misuse.

   Furthermore, unresolved emotional traumas or unfavorable childhood experiences can trap the nervous system in a hyper- or hyperarousal state, leading to dysregulation.

4. **Genetics:** A dysregulated neurological system can be inherited by an individual. People who have specific gene variants may be more prone to stress and anxiety, which can lead to nervous system dysregulation.

5. **Lifestyle Factors:** Unhealthy eating habits, inactivity, and insufficient sleep can all impair your nervous system's ability to operate normally. In particular, stimulants like alcohol and coffee are drugs that overstimulate the neural system and cause dysregulation.

6. **Underlying Health Conditions:** Nervous system dysregulation can be exacerbated by several illnesses, including autoimmune

diseases, fibromyalgia, chronic fatigue syndrome, and hormone imbalances.

Nutritionally speaking, the nervous system can become dysregulated due to a lack of specific nutrients, such as magnesium, omega-3 fatty acids, B vitamins, and others, which are necessary for the nervous system to function properly.

7. **Environmental Factors:** The nervous system's ability to operate properly might be adversely affected by exposure to environmental pollutants such as heavy metals, pesticides, mold, and some chemicals. Dysregulation can also be caused by stressors like excessive levels of stress at work or noise pollution.

To treat the problem and start along the path toward a regulated neurological system, it is adviceable to understand these factors. It's also critical to remember that these variables frequently interact, and a dysregulated neurological system usually has multiple contributing elements. Let's talk about the typical signs and symptoms of a dysregulated neural system now that we are aware of the causes of dysregulation.

Risk factors that may cause variety of symptoms, include the following:

- Persistent anxiety or stress

- Exhaustion

- persistent discomfort

- elevated blood pressure

- Immunological systems and gut dysfunctions

- Mood disorders

- Anxiety-related disorders

- PTSD, or post-traumatic stress disorder

- disruptions to sleep

- difficulties with the senses

- Changes in mood

- Intolerance

- Weary

- digestive problems

- Headaches

- headaches

- The fibromyalgia

- Hypersensitivity

- Inhalation

- Diabetes

- Cancer and rheumatoid arthritis

Who is at risk for nervous system dysregulation?

Almost everybody is susceptible to a dysregulated neurological system, primarily because of our increasingly demanding everyday lives. For many of us, everyday life now includes rush hour traffic, financial strains, and rigid work schedules, which foster chronic stress.

Perfectionism is one trait that can increase your risk of having a dysregulated neurological system, as does excessive stress at work or school. There are a few other things that could make you more vulnerable:

- Past experiences with emotional or psychological abuse

- Past experiences with catastrophic incidents or PTSD (post-traumatic stress disorder)

- Past instances of tiredness or burnout

- Concussions and traumatic brain injuries

- imbalances in hormones

- metabolic illnesses, such as diabetes

You may find answers to your persistent health issues by becoming aware of your hazards and the process by which a dysregulated neural system develops. Thankfully, a dysregulated neurological system may always be healed, even if things appear unchangeable.

Consequences of a dysregulated nervous system

A dysregulated neural system can result in behaviors that are detrimental to leading a healthy, balanced life, as well as mental health problems including anxiety, depression, sleeplessness, and difficulty focusing and remembering things. These behaviors include:

tense interactions with coworkers, lovers, friends, or family

Bad decisions made in life (such as abusing substances or engaging in addictive behaviors) are a result of attempting to escape the discomfort brought on by the dysregulation of our neurological systems and the resulting symptoms of mental illness.

acting in a way that is unhealthy, shortsighted, and harmful to both ourselves and other people because our prefrontal cortex—the area of the brain that is more organized, rational, and planning—is not in charge of our thoughts and behaviors, which are controlled by our limbic system—the more primitive, emotional, and reflexive part of the brain.

A dysregulated neural system may cause information processing and response issues in the brain. Anomalous patterns of physiological, physical, and cognitive reactions can arise from malfunctions in the sympathetic or parasympathetic nervous systems.

Hyper- and hyperarousal are among the most common effects of dysregulation. An elevated fight-or-flight reaction, characterized by feelings of rage, impulsivity, racing thoughts, and defensiveness, is referred to as hyperarousal. Reduced reactivity and a freeze-or-fawn behavioral reaction are signs of hyperarousal. People in this state feel numb, have more depressive moods, have trouble thinking clearly, and shut down. If one frequently experiences these extremes in mood, it may be a sign that self-regulation and mindfulness are needed, along with treatment and knowledge of the causes of dysregulation.

Studies reveal that adolescents and teenagers with dysregulated neural systems frequently experience emotional dysregulation, sleep disturbances, and digestive disorders. A dysregulated neurological system can also result in the following problems if left unchecked:

Mood swings, anxiety, tension, depression, and irritability are examples of psychological symptoms.

Physical signs and symptoms: headaches, immune system compromise, persistent pain, tense muscles, and sleeplessness

Cognitive symptoms include trouble concentrating, being easily overwhelmed, having memory issues, and being too sensitive to stimuli.

Summing Up

Nervous system dysregulation is a condition where the sympathetic nervous system (SNS) is activated more frequently than usual, leading to a loss of control and deterioration of the body. Factors contributing to this dysregulation include psychological aspects such as trauma and stress, lifestyle and biochemical elements, and underlying health conditions.

Challenges include chronic stress, which can lead to overreaction and hypervigilance, and adverse childhood experiences (ACEs), which can affect the nervous system's development and lead to dysregulation. Genetics can also play a role in this condition, with individuals with specific gene variants being more prone to stress and anxiety. Lifestyle factors, such as unhealthy eating habits, inactivity, and insufficient sleep, can impair the nervous system's ability to operate normally.

Underlying health conditions, such as autoimmune diseases, fibromyalgia, chronic fatigue syndrome, and hormone imbalances, can exacerbate nervous system dysregulation. Nutritionally, the nervous system can become dysregulated due to a lack of specific nutrients. Environmental factors, such as heavy metals, pesticides, mold, and chemicals, can also adversely affect the nervous system's ability to operate properly.

To treat a dysregulated neurological system, it is essential to understand these factors and their interactions. Symptoms of dysregulation may include persistent anxiety, exhaustion, discomfort, elevated blood pressure, mood disorders, anxiety-related disorders, PTSD, sleep disruptions, sense-related difficulties, intolerance, fatigue, digestive problems, headaches, fibromyalgia, hypersensitivity, inhalation, diabetes, and cancer and rheumatoid arthritis.

Nervous system dysregulation is a common issue in today's demanding lives, often resulting from factors such as perfectionism, excessive stress, past emotional or psychological abuse, PTSD, burnout, traumatic brain injuries, hormone imbalances, and metabolic illnesses. Dysregulated neural systems can lead to negative behaviors, such as anxiety, depression, sleeplessness, and difficulty focusing and remembering. These behaviors can lead to unhealthy decisions, such as substance abuse or addictive behaviors. Dysregulated neural systems can cause abnormal patterns of physiological, physical, and cognitive reactions, leading to hyperarousal and other symptoms. Adolescents and teenagers with dysregulated neural systems often experience emotional dysregulation, sleep disturbances, and digestive disorders. Unchecked, these symptoms can lead to mood swings, anxiety, tension, depression, irritability, physical symptoms like headaches, immune system compromise, persistent pain, tense muscles, sleeplessness, and cognitive symptoms like difficulty concentrating, overwhelmingness, memory issues, and sensitivity to stimuli.

CHAPTER 3: Test and Diagnosis

Dysregulated nervous system test

A dysregulated nervous system can manifest in various ways, making it essential to identify the signs and symptoms. Here are some common indicators:

- **Heightened sensitivity to stimuli**: You may experience increased irritability, anxiety, difficulty concentrating, or trouble focusing. You might feel overwhelmed or easily triggered by everyday situations.

- **Over reactivity**: You may overreact to perceived threats, even if there is no rational danger. This can lead to emotional and physical responses that take hours or days to recover from.

- **Oversensitivity**: You may be overly sensitive to certain sounds, smells, or textures, which can be distressing and affect your daily life.

- **Chronic stress**: You may experience prolonged periods of stress, leading to burnout, anxiety, or depression.

- **Sleep disturbances**: You may struggle with insomnia, restlessness, or difficulty falling asleep due to an overactive nervous system.

- **Physical symptoms**: You may experience chronic pain, muscle tension, or digestive issues, which can be linked to a dysregulated nervous system.

- **Mood swings**: You may experience rapid mood shifts, from feeling calm to anxious or irritable, without an apparent reason.

- **Brain fog**: You may struggle with concentration, memory, or decision-making due to an overactive or underactive nervous system.

To identify if you have a dysregulated nervous system, ask yourself:

- Do you experience frequent feelings of anxiety, stress, or overwhelm?

- Do you have trouble sleeping or experience insomnia?

- Do you feel irritable, sensitive, or reactive to certain stimuli?

- Do you experience chronic pain, muscle tension, or digestive issues?

- Do you struggle with concentration, memory, or decision-making?

If you have identify with several of these signs and symptoms, it may be beneficial to consult with a healthcare professional for further evaluation and guidance on rebalancing your nervous system.

What is the diagnosis of the dysregulated nervous system?

Here are some potential diagnoses related to a dysregulated nervous system:

1. **Nervous System Dysregulation**: A state of imbalance between the sympathetic and parasympathetic nervous systems, leading to symptoms such as feeling overwhelmed, anxious, or stressed.

2. **Autonomic Dysfunction**: A condition where the autonomic nervous system, which regulates various bodily functions, is impaired, leading to symptoms such as dizziness, lightheadedness, or changes in heart rate.
3. **Neurodevelopmental Disorders**: Conditions such as autism, ADHD, or sensory processing disorder, which can be related to nervous system dysregulation.
4. **Chronic Stress**: Prolonged exposure to stress can lead to a dysregulated nervous system, causing symptoms such as anxiety, depression, or burnout.
5. **Post-Traumatic Stress Disorder (PTSD)**: A condition that can develop after a traumatic event, characterized by symptoms such as flashbacks, nightmares, and hypervigilance, which can be related to nervous system dysregulation.
6. **Anxiety Disorders**: Conditions such as generalized anxiety disorder, panic disorder, or social anxiety disorder, can be related to nervous system dysregulation.
7. **Depression**: A mood disorder characterized by feelings of sadness, hopelessness, and loss of interest in activities, which can be related to nervous system dysregulation.

8. **Chronic Pain**: Persistent pain can be related to nervous system dysregulation, which can be caused by various factors such as inflammation, trauma, or chronic stress.

9. **Fibromyalgia**: A condition characterized by widespread muscle pain, fatigue, and sleep disturbances, which can be related to nervous system dysregulation.

10. **Hypervigilance**: A state of increased alertness and awareness, which can be related to nervous system dysregulation and can be seen in conditions such as PTSD or anxiety disorders.

1. **Nervous System Dysregulation**

Understanding Nervous System Dysregulation

Nervous system dysregulation refers to a malfunction or imbalance within the nervous system, which affects its normal functioning and capacity to regulate responses to stimuli. This can manifest in various ways, ranging from physiological to emotional and cognitive disturbances.

Signs and Symptoms

- Some common signs and symptoms of nervous system dysregulation include:

- Heightened sensitivity to stimuli

- Increased irritability

- Difficulty concentrating or focusing

- Trouble sleeping or insomnia

- Chronic pain or muscle tension

- Digestive problems

- Fatigue or exhaustion

- Anxiety or panic attacks

- Mood swings or emotional instability

- Difficulty regulating emotions

- Increased stress response

- Decreased resilience to stress

Causes

Nervous system dysregulation can be caused by a variety of factors, including:

- Chronic stress or trauma

- Poor diet or nutrition

- Lack of exercise or physical activity

- Sleep deprivation or disorders

- Substance abuse or addiction

- Medical conditions or illnesses

- Genetic predisposition

- Environmental toxins or pollutants

- Lack of social support or connection

- Rebalancing Techniques

Fortunately, many techniques can help rebalance and regulate the nervous system, including:

- Deep breathing exercises

- Progressive muscle relaxation

- Meditation and mindfulness practices

- Yoga or tai chi

- Exercise or physical activity

- Aromatherapy or essential oils

- Herbal remedies or supplements

- Cognitive-behavioral therapy (CBT)

- Mindfulness-based stress reduction (MBSR)

- Biofeedback therapy

- Neurofeedback therapy

Importance of Nervous System Regulation

Nervous system regulation is essential for maintaining overall health and well-being. A dysregulated nervous system can lead to a range of negative consequences, including:

- Chronic stress and anxiety

- Mood disorders or depression

- Sleep disturbances or insomnia

- Chronic pain or fatigue

- Decreased resilience to stress

- Impaired cognitive function or memory

- A higher risk of disease or illness

By understanding the signs and symptoms of nervous system dysregulation and implementing rebalancing techniques, individuals can take steps to promote nervous system regulation and improve overall health and well-being.

2. Autonomic Dysfunction

Autonomic dysfunction is a condition where the autonomic nervous system (ANS), which controls various involuntary functions of the body, such as heart rate, blood pressure, digestion, and sweating, does not function properly. This can lead to a range of symptoms and disorders, including orthostatic hypotension, postural tachycardia syndrome (POTS), and changes in gastrointestinal and urinary habits.

The autonomic nervous system is a complex network of nerves that work together to regulate various bodily functions, such as:

- Blood pressure and heart rate

- Body temperature

- Digestion

- Bladder and bowel function

- Sweating

- Pupil size

- Blood vessel constriction and dilation

When the ANS is damaged or dysfunctional, it can lead to a range of symptoms, including:

- Orthostatic hypotension: a sudden drop in blood pressure when standing up

- Postural tachycardia syndrome (POTS): a rapid increase in heart rate when standing up

- Gastroparesis: slowed or stopped movement of food from the stomach to the small intestine

- Gastroparesis can lead to malabsorption of glucose and insulin, making it difficult to manage blood sugar levels

- Bladder and bowel dysfunction

- Changes in sweating and pupil size

- Fluctuations in blood pressure

Autonomic dysfunction can occur as a primary condition or as a secondary complication of other diseases, such as Parkinson's disease, diabetes, and multiple sclerosis. Treatment for autonomic dysfunction typically involves managing symptoms and addressing underlying causes, as well as lifestyle changes such as increasing fluid intake, avoiding dehydration, and exercising regularly.

3. Neurodevelopmental Disorders

Neurodevelopmental disorders are a group of conditions that affect the brain and nervous system's development and function. These disorders can impact various aspects of a person's life, including social, cognitive, and emotional functioning. Neurodevelopmental disorders can be caused by a combination of genetic and environmental factors and can manifest in different ways depending on the individual.

Some common neurodevelopmental disorders include:

- Autism Spectrum Disorder (ASD)

- Attention Deficit Hyperactivity Disorder (ADHD)

- Intellectual Disability

- Learning Disabilities

- Neurodevelopmental Motor Disorders, including Tic Disorders

- Specific Learning Disorders

- Nonverbal Learning Disorder (NLD)

These disorders can affect anyone, regardless of their background or environment. They can also co-occur with other conditions, such as mental health disorders or physical disabilities.

Neurodevelopmental disorders can be diagnosed and treated by a variety of healthcare professionals, including psychologists, psychiatrists, and neurologists. Treatment options may include behavioral therapy, medication, and accommodations to help individuals with neurodevelopmental disorders manage their symptoms and improve their functioning.

4. Chronic Stress

Chronic stress is a prolonged and constant feeling of stress that can negatively affect one's health if left untreated. It is different from acute stress, which is a reaction to a specific event. Chronic stress is a consistent sense of feeling pressured and overwhelmed over a long period. It can be caused by everyday pressures of family and work or by traumatic situations. The body experiences stressful situations so frequently that it doesn't have a chance to activate its relaxation response, so the mind and body may not recover.

Chronic stress is not tied to a particular moment, but rather is a result of a significant persistent problem or a combination of interchangeable problems over some time. It can be episodic, meaning a person experiences it over a long time but inconsistently, or it can be continuous, feeling stressed throughout their life to the point where feeling stressed becomes a normal state of being.

Chronic stress can have severe mental and physical health complications, such as a consistent feeling of being under pressure or overwhelmed, which can lead to a range of symptoms including anxiety, depression, and burnout. It can also affect the immune system and damage multiple organs and tissues over time.

5. Post-Traumatic Stress Disorder (PTSD)

Post-Traumatic Stress Disorder (PTSD) is a psychiatric disorder that may occur in people who have experienced or witnessed a traumatic event, a series of events, or a set of circumstances that is emotionally or physically harmful or life-threatening. This can include events such as combat, natural disasters, car accidents, sexual assault, or other traumatic experiences.

PTSD can cause a range of symptoms, including:

- Disturbing thoughts, feelings, or dreams related to the event

- Mental or physical distress to trauma-related cues

- Efforts to avoid trauma-related situations

- Increased fight-or-flight response

PTSD can also lead to complications, such as:

- Suicide

- Cardiac, respiratory, musculoskeletal, gastrointestinal, and immunological disorders

The duration of PTSD can vary, but it is typically characterized by symptoms that last for more than one month. PTSD is often caused by exposure to a traumatic event, and the diagnostic method is based on symptoms.

Treatment for PTSD typically involves counseling, medication, and

MDMA-assisted psychotherapy. Selective serotonin reuptake inhibitors (SSRIs) are also commonly used to treat PTSD. The incidence of PTSD varies, with a lifetime risk of 8.7% and a 12-month risk of 3.5% in the United States.

6. Anxiety disorders

Anxiety disorders are a type of mental health condition characterized by excessive and persistent feelings of fear, worry, and anxiety that are not proportional to the actual situation. These disorders can interfere with daily life, causing significant distress and impairment in social, occupational, or other areas of functioning.

Anxiety disorders can manifest in various forms, including:

- Generalized anxiety disorder (GAD): is characterized by excessive and persistent worry about everyday things, such as work, finances, or health.

- Panic disorder: characterized by recurring panic attacks, which are sudden episodes of intense fear or discomfort that peak within minutes and include physical symptoms such as a racing heart, sweating, and trembling.

- Social anxiety disorder (SAD): characterized by excessive fear or anxiety in social or performance situations, such as public speaking, meeting new people, or being the center of attention.

- Specific phobias: characterized by an excessive or irrational fear of a specific object, situation, or activity, such as spiders, heights, or enclosed spaces.

- Post-traumatic stress disorder (PTSD): is characterized by symptoms that occur after a person experiences a traumatic event, such as a natural disaster, assault, or military combat.

Common symptoms of anxiety disorders include:

- Persistent and excessive worry or fear

- Restlessness, feeling on edge, or irritability

- Fatigue, difficulty concentrating, or insomnia

- Rapid heartbeat, sweating, trembling, or other physical symptoms

- Avoidance of situations or activities due to fear or anxiety

Anxiety disorders can be caused by a combination of genetic, environmental, and psychological factors, including:

- Genetic predisposition

- Childhood trauma or abuse

- Family history of anxiety disorders

- Environmental stressors, such as work or financial stress

- Brain chemistry imbalances

Treatment for anxiety disorders typically involves a combination of therapy, such as cognitive-behavioral therapy (CBT), and medication, such as antidepressants or benzodiazepines. Lifestyle changes, such as regular exercise, relaxation techniques, and stress management, can also help manage symptoms.

7. Depression

Depression is a disorder of the brain that is more than just a feeling of being "down in the dumps" or "blue" for a few days. It is a serious mental illness that can affect all aspects of life, including relationships with family, friends, and community, and can result in problems at school and work. Depression can happen to anyone, and it is estimated that more than 20 million people in the United States have depression.

Depression is characterized by a persistent feeling of sadness, hopelessness, and a lack of interest in activities that were once enjoyed. It can also cause changes in appetite, sleep, energy levels, and concentration. Depression can be caused by a combination of genetic, environmental, and psychological factors, and it can be treated with a combination of therapy, medication, and lifestyle changes.

Some common depression symptoms include:

- Feeling sad, empty, or hopeless

- Loss of interest in activities that were once enjoyed

- Changes in appetite or sleep patterns

- Fatigue or loss of energy

- Difficulty concentrating or making decisions

- Irritability or restlessness

- Physical symptoms such as headaches, stomachaches, or muscle pain

Depression is distinct from regular mood changes and feelings in everyday life. It is a serious condition that requires professional treatment and support.

8. Chronic pain

Chronic pain is a type of pain that lasts for more than three months, or in some cases, beyond the normal healing time. It is different from acute pain, which is a normal response to an injury or illness and typically subsides once the underlying cause is treated or healed. Chronic pain can be a persistent and debilitating condition that can significantly impact a person's quality of life, daily activities, and overall well-being.

Chronic pain can be caused by a variety of factors, including:

- High blood sugar

- Cancer

- Genetic disorders in neural differentiation

- Tissue damage

- Neurological disorders

- Viral diseases

It can also be triggered by a range of factors, such as:

- Heavy and irregular sports or physical activities

- Injuries or illnesses that do not fully heal

- Underlying medical conditions, such as diabetes, cancer, or heart disease

- Psychological factors, such as depression, anxiety, or stress

Symptoms of chronic pain can vary widely and may include:

- Pain that persists or worsens over time

- Pain that is constant or intermittent

- Pain that is localized to a specific area of the body or widespread

- Pain that is accompanied by other symptoms, such as fatigue, sleep disturbances, or mood changes

Chronic pain can be managed through a combination of medications, therapies, and lifestyle changes. Treatment options may include:

- Non-opioid medications, such as ibuprofen or acetaminophen

- Opioid medications, such as morphine or codeine

- Alternative therapies, such as physical therapy, acupuncture, or massage

- Lifestyle changes, such as exercise, stress management, or relaxation techniques

- Cognitive-behavioral therapy to address psychological factors

It is essential to work with a healthcare provider to develop a personalized treatment plan to manage chronic pain and improve quality of life.

9. Fibromyalgia

Fibromyalgia is a chronic (long-lasting) disorder that causes pain and tenderness throughout the body, as well as fatigue and trouble sleeping. Scientists do not fully understand what causes it, but people with the disorder have an increased sensitivity to pain.

There is no cure for fibromyalgia, but doctors and other healthcare providers can help manage and treat the symptoms. Treatment typically involves a combination of exercise or other movement therapies, psychological and behavioral therapy, and medications.

Who Gets Fibromyalgia?

Anyone can get fibromyalgia, but more women get it than men. It can affect people of any age, even children, but it usually starts in middle age, and the chance of having it increases as you get older. It affects people of all racial and ethnic backgrounds.

If you have other diseases, especially rheumatic diseases, mood disorders, or conditions that cause pain, you may be more likely to have fibromyalgia. These diseases include:

- Rheumatoid arthritis.

- Systemic lupus erythematosus (commonly called lupus).

- Ankylosing spondylitis.

- Osteoarthritis.

- Depression or anxiety.

- Chronic back pain.

- Irritable bowel syndrome.

Fibromyalgia tends to run in families, and some scientists believe that certain genes could make you more likely to develop it. However, the disorder also occurs in people with no family history of the disorder.

Symptoms of Fibromyalgia

Fibromyalgia's main symptoms include:

- Chronic, widespread pain throughout the body or in multiple areas. Pain is often felt in the arms, legs, head, chest, abdomen, back, and buttocks. People often describe it as aching, burning, or throbbing.

- Fatigue or an overwhelming feeling of being tired.

- Trouble sleeping.

Other symptoms may include:

- Muscle and joint stiffness.

- Tenderness to touch.

- Numbness or tingling in the arms and legs.

- Problems with concentrating, thinking clearly, and memory (sometimes called "fibro fog").

- Increased sensitivity to light, noise, odors, and temperature.

- Digestive issues, such as bloating or constipation.

Causes of Fibromyalgia

The cause of fibromyalgia is not known, but studies show that people with the disorder have an increased sensitivity to pain, so they feel pain when others do not. In people with fibromyalgia, brain imaging studies, and other research have uncovered evidence of altered signaling in neural pathways that transmit and receive pain. These changes may also contribute to the fatigue, sleep troubles, and "fibro fog" issues that many people with the disorder experience.

Fibromyalgia tends to run in families, so genetic factors are likely to contribute to the disorder. However, little is known for sure about the specific genes involved. Researchers believe that environmental (nongenetic) factors also play a role in a person's risk of developing the disorder. These environmental triggers may include having a disease that causes pain, such as rheumatoid arthritis, or mental health problems, such as anxiety or depression.

10. Hypervigilance

Hypervigilance is a state of increased alertness. If you're in a state of hypervigilance, you're extremely sensitive to your surroundings. It can make you feel like you're alert to any hidden dangers, whether from other people or the environment. Often, though, these dangers are not real.

Hypervigilance can be a symptom of mental health conditions, such as:

- post-traumatic stress disorder (PTSD)

- anxiety disorders

- schizophrenia

These can all cause your brain and your body to constantly be on high alert. Hypervigilance can hurt your life. It can affect how you interact with and view others, or it may encourage paranoia.

Hypervigilance symptoms

Hypervigilance can be accompanied by physical, behavioral, emotional, and mental symptoms:

Physical symptoms

Physical symptoms may resemble those of anxiety. These may include:

- sweating

- Fast heart rate

- fast, shallow breathing

- Over time, this constant state of alertness can cause fatigue and exhaustion.

Behavioral symptoms

Behavioral symptoms include jumpy reflexes and fast, knee-jerk reactions to your environment. If you're hypervigilant, you may overreact if you hear a loud bang or if you misunderstand a coworker's statement as rude. These reactions may be violent or hostile in an apparent attempt to defend yourself.

Emotional symptoms

The emotional symptoms of hypervigilance can be severe. These can include:

- increased, severe anxiety

- fear

- panic

- worrying that can become persistent

You may fear judgment from others, or you may judge others extremely harshly. This may develop into black-and-white thinking in which you find things either right or wrong. You can also become emotionally withdrawn. You may experience mood swings or outbursts of emotion.

Mental symptoms

Paranoia can be a mental symptom of hypervigilance. This may be accompanied by rationalization to justify the hypervigilance. It can also be difficult for those who experience frequent hypervigilance, like those with PTSD, to sleep well.

Long-term symptoms

If you experience recurring hypervigilance, you may start to develop behaviors to calm your anxiety or counteract perceived threats. If you fear assault or danger, for example, you may start carrying a concealed weapon. If you have severe social anxiety, you may rely on daydreaming or non-participation in events. These symptoms can result in social isolation and damaged relationships.

Causes of hypervigilance

Hypervigilance can be caused by different mental health conditions:

Anxiety: Anxiety is one of the most common causes of hypervigilance. If you have generalized anxiety disorder, you might be hypervigilant in new situations or environments that you're unfamiliar with.

If you have social anxiety, you may be hypervigilant in the presence of others, especially new people or people you don't trust.

PTSD: PTSD is another common cause of hypervigilance. PTSD can cause you to be tense. You may constantly scan the area for perceived threats.

Schizophrenia: Schizophrenia can also cause hypervigilance. Hypervigilance can worsen other symptoms of the condition, such as paranoia or hallucinations.

Common triggers

Some common triggers can cause or contribute to episodes of hypervigilance. These include:

- feeling trapped or claustrophobic

- feeling abandoned

- hearing loud noises (especially if they're -sudden or emotionally charged), which can -include yelling, arguments, and sudden bangs

- anticipating pain, fear, or judgment

- feeling judged or unwelcome

- feeling physical pain

- feeling emotional distress

- being reminded of past traumas

- being around random, chaotic behaviors of others

Summing Up

Dysregulated nervous system tests are essential for identifying signs and symptoms of a dysfunctional nervous system. Common indicators include increased sensitivity to stimuli, overreactivity, oversensitivity, chronic stress, sleep disturbances, physical symptoms, mood swings, and brain fog. To identify a dysregulated nervous system, ask yourself if you experience frequent feelings of anxiety, stress, or overwhelm, trouble sleeping or insomnia, irritability, sensitivity to certain stimuli, chronic pain, muscle tension, digestive issues, and difficulty with concentration, memory, or decision-making.

Diagnosis of a dysregulated nervous system includes Nervous System Dysregulation, Autonomic Dysfunction, Neurodevelopmental Disorders, Chronic Stress, Post-Traumatic Stress Disorder (PTSD), Anxiety Disorders,

Depression, Chronic Pain, Fibromyalgia, and Hypervigilance. Causes of nervous system dysregulation can include chronic stress, poor diet, lack of exercise, sleep deprivation, substance abuse, medical conditions, genetic predisposition, environmental toxins, and lack of social support.

Rebalancing techniques can help rebalance and regulate the nervous system, including deep breathing exercises, progressive muscle relaxation, meditation and mindfulness practices, yoga, exercise, aromatherapy, herbal remedies, cognitive-behavioral therapy (CBT), mindfulness-based stress reduction (MBSR), biofeedback therapy, and neurofeedback therapy.

Nervous system regulation is essential for maintaining overall health and well-being, as a dysregulated nervous system can lead to negative consequences such as chronic stress and anxiety, mood disorders or depression, sleep disturbances or insomnia, chronic pain or fatigue, decreased resilience to stress, impaired cognitive function or memory, and a higher risk of disease or illness. By understanding these signs and symptoms and implementing rebalancing techniques, individuals can promote nervous system regulation and improve overall health and well-being.

Autonomic dysfunction is a condition where the autonomic nervous system (ANS) fails to function properly, leading to symptoms such as orthostatic hypotension, postural tachycardia syndrome (POTS), and changes in gastrointestinal and urinary habits. It can occur as a primary condition or as a secondary complication of other diseases. Treatment for autonomic dysfunction typically involves managing symptoms and addressing underlying causes, as well as lifestyle changes.

Neurodevelopmental disorders affect the brain and nervous system's development and function, impacting social, cognitive, and emotional functioning. Common neurodevelopmental disorders include Autism Spectrum Disorder (ASD), Attention Deficit Hyperactivity Disorder (ADHD), Intellectual Disability, Learning Disabilities, Neurodevelopmental Motor Disorders, Specific Learning Disorders, and Nonverbal Learning Disorder (NLD). These disorders can affect anyone, regardless of their background or environment, and can co-occur with other conditions.

Chronic stress is a prolonged and constant feeling of pressure and overwhelm over a long period, caused by everyday pressures or traumatic situations. It can have severe mental and physical health complications, such as anxiety, depression, and burnout, and can damage multiple organs and tissues over time.

Post-Traumatic Stress Disorder (PTSD) is a psychiatric disorder resulting from experiencing or witnessing a traumatic event or series of events. It can cause disturbing thoughts, feelings, dreams, mental or physical distress, attempts to avoid trauma-related situations, and increased fight-or-flight response. Treatment for PTSD typically involves counseling, medication, and MDMA-assisted psychotherapy.

Anxiety disorders are mental health conditions characterized by excessive and persistent feelings of fear, worry, and anxiety that are not proportional to the actual situation. They can manifest in various forms, such as generalized anxiety disorder (GAD), panic disorder, social anxiety disorder (SAD), specific phobias, and post-traumatic stress disorder (PTSD). Common symptoms include persistent worry, restlessness, fatigue, difficulty concentrating, insomnia, and avoidance of situations or activities due to fear or anxiety.

Depression is a serious mental illness that affects all aspects of life, including relationships with family, friends, and community. It can be caused by genetic, environmental, and psychological factors and can be treated with a combination of therapy, medication, and lifestyle changes. Common symptoms include feeling sad, hopeless, loss of interest in activities, changes in appetite or sleep patterns, fatigue, difficulty concentrating, irritability, and physical symptoms.

Chronic pain is a persistent and debilitating condition that can significantly impact a person's quality of life, daily activities, and overall well-being. It can be caused by various factors, such as high blood sugar, cancer, genetic disorders in neural differentiation, tissue damage, neurological disorders, and viral diseases. Treatment options may include non-opioid medications, opioid medications, alternative therapies, lifestyle changes, and cognitive-behavioral therapy.

Fibromyalgia is a chronic disorder that causes pain, tenderness, fatigue, and trouble sleeping.

Although there is no cure for fibromyalgia, doctors and healthcare providers can help manage and treat symptoms through exercise, psychological and behavioral therapy, and medications.

Fibromyalgia is a condition that affects people of all racial and ethnic backgrounds, with more women experiencing it than men. It typically starts in middle age and increases as individuals get older. People with other diseases, such as rheumatic diseases, mood disorders, or conditions that cause pain, may be more likely to have fibromyalgia. The disorder can run in families, and some scientists believe certain genes could make individuals more likely to develop it.

Symptoms of fibromyalgia include chronic, widespread pain throughout the body, fatigue, trouble sleeping, muscle and joint stiffness, tenderness to touch, numbness or tingling, problems with concentration, thinking clearly, and memory (sometimes called "fibro fog"), increased sensitivity to light, noise, odors, and temperature, and digestive issues.

The cause of fibromyalgia is unknown, but studies show that people with the disorder have an increased sensitivity to pain, which may contribute to fatigue, sleep troubles, and "fibro fog" issues. Genetic factors are likely to contribute to the disorder, but environmental factors, such as having a disease that causes pain or mental health problems, also play a role in a person's risk of developing the disorder.

Hypervigilance is a state of increased alertness, often accompanied by physical, behavioral, emotional, and mental symptoms. Causes of hypervigilance include anxiety, PTSD, schizophrenia, and common triggers like feeling trapped or claustrophobic, abandoned, hearing loud noises, anticipating pain, fear, judgment, being judged or unwelcome, feeling physical pain, emotional distress, being reminded of past traumas, and being around random, chaotic behaviors of others.

CHAPTER 4: Treatment for Nervous System Dysregulation

Methods for Restoring a Nervous System That Is Dysregulated

Do you experience anxiety, burnout, or trauma as someone with a sensitive nervous system? Then you are not by yourself. These are typical indicators of a dysregulated neurological system, which can be brought on by several things, including sleep deprivation, traumatic events, and long-term stress.

Fortunately, there are lots of things you can do to enhance your quality of life and aid in the healing of your neurological system. We shall describe 47 techniques in this book that are helpful for individuals with dysregulated neural systems. These techniques can raise energy levels, lessen stress and anxiety, enhance the quality of sleep, and advance general health and well-being. So continue reading if you're prepared to begin treating your dysregulated neurological system!

I hope that these activities will be beneficial to you and lead to a healthier and happier existence.

Which techniques work best for treating a neurological system that is dysregulated?

When it comes to enumerating the greatest ways to cure a dysregulated neural system, there isn't a single, universal solution. Based on your neurological system's particular sensitivity and level of dysregulation, some basic recommendations can be made. For instance, lifestyle modifications like better eating, consistent exercise, and good sleep hygiene can benefit everyone, but they're more important for those with high sensitivity. Body-mind exercises like yoga, meditation, or breathwork may be helpful to others. Others might benefit from visiting a therapist and/or using supplements to aid their nervous system. In the end, it's critical to try out several strategies and determine which ones are most effective for you.

1. **7–9 hours of undisturbed, deep sleep**

   Uninterrupted, deep sleep is essential for general wellness. The majority of people are aware of the significance of sleep, but they might not understand how vital it is to general health and well-being. Others experience periods of worry and insomnia. The body has an opportunity to rest and heal itself when we sleep. During this period, the brain also purges itself of any poisons that may have accumulated during the day. You may experience sleep issues, such as difficulty falling asleep or waking up during the night if your neurological system is dysregulated. You can do a lot of things to improve your quality of sleep, so don't worry!

By minimizing our exposure to light after sunset or by exposing our eyes to the sun in the morning, we can enhance our sleep. Don't eat two to three hours before bed. Find out how your circadian rhythm influences your sleep cycles.

2. Deep Breathing

Deep breathing is one way to support the neurological system and blood oxygenation. The muscle that divides the chest cavity from the abdominal cavity is called the diaphragm. One of the simplest ways to relax your nervous system is to breathe deeply. To test this, take a seat in a comfortable position and expand your chest and abdomen while inhaling through your nose. Take a deep breath out of your mouth and prolong your exhalation. When you do that, attempt to focus just on the airflow that passes through your abdomen, lungs, and nose before returning via your mouth. If you find doing so helpful, shut your eyes and place your palm on your chest to feel its expansion.

3. **Moderate exercise, such as walking, dancing, and running**

Exercise is recognized to be beneficial to the body, but what about moderate exercise? Research has indicated that even a modest amount of movement might benefit the nervous system. Developing an embodiment practice could help you develop body awareness. Physical movement also enables you to balance dysregulation and release stress. Choose a fun activity to engage in, and afterward, get the endorphin rush. You can join a running group or take dance classes if you need more incentive. Who knows, perhaps you'll find a new interest and meet people.

4. **Co-regulation in a safe relationship with a loved one**

In a safe and harmonious partnership, co-regulation takes place. We can simultaneously control our nervous systems when we establish a connection with a loved one who is in a regulated state through touch, breath, or vocal mirroring. This aids in our transition from a dysregulated condition. Numerous advantages of co-regulation have been demonstrated, such as less anxiety and enhanced sleep quality. Co-regulating with a loved one gives us access to an effective technique for stress reduction and well-being enhancement. Stress is reduced and we feel more secure when we are in a healthy relationship where we can rely on the other person.

5. Qi Gong, Tai Chi, and Yoga

It has been demonstrated that ancient techniques including yoga, tai chi, and qigong can effectively relax the nervous system. These simple exercises can be readily introduced into a hectic lifestyle, while also helping to develop bodily balance and relaxation. They do provide a great means of lowering stress and enhancing general wellness. By using these approaches, you can become more conscious of your feelings. You can learn to identify emotions as they arise if you can identify the tension in your body. Yoga teaches proper breathing, as well as developing the peripheral nervous system. When it comes to yoga styles, you have an abundance of options.

6. Chanting and singing

Singing and chanting are two powerful methods for calming the nervous system. Chanting is one vocalization technique that is frequently employed in religious or spiritual activities. It entails repeatedly using the same word or phrase. Repetition like this can aid in mental clarity and attention. Singing is another excellent way to calm the nervous system.

Chanting and singing trigger the vagus nerve and cause your respiration to slow down. Vocal stimulation is one of the shortest routes from fight-or-flight (dysregulation) to rest and digest. Even if you only sing at home, singing may be a powerful tool for communicating feelings. How about throwing a small concert for yourself?

7. Strolling with bare feet on the grass, beach, and in nature

It is beneficial to go barefoot on unpaved surfaces to help calm your nervous system. Your feet absorb electrons from the earth, which helps you unwind. It helps to ground your nervous system by allowing you to establish a connection between your feet and the soil's surface. Nature's calming effects on the human mind have been scientifically proven. According to a study, it may aid with stress reduction, inflammation, heart rate variability, improved sleep, cortisol management, and autonomic nervous system balance. Our feet might benefit from a good massage when we stroll along the beach.

8. Massage

A massage is not just about unwinding. It has been demonstrated to benefit the neurological system, enhancing blood flow and assisting in the decrease of stress-related chemicals. It has also been demonstrated that massage helps to lessen pain and inflammation. One way to stimulate the parasympathetic division is through massage therapy. Massage therapy helps the body regain equilibrium, which promotes better sleep and focus. Your body may flow easily with oxygen and blood after receiving a decent massage. It also helps to relax your muscles, which become excessively tight when you're under a lot of stress. You'll notice that you become more at ease and joyful when your body and mind are at ease.

9. Smells

Among the strongest senses is the smell. It can elicit feelings and memories, as well as have unforeseen behavioral effects. For instance, we may feel more alert when we smell coffee, yet we may feel hungry when we smell freshly baked bread. Therefore, it should come as no surprise that our neurological system and sense of smell are strongly related. Numerous studies demonstrate how aromas can reduce stress. Even a single whiff of scents like coffee beans and essential oils has been demonstrated to lower brain stress signals.

10. Resting and relaxation without screen time or obligations

The majority of us are constantly stimulated by our electronics. Even though unplugging can be challenging, it's crucial to set aside some time for leisure and relaxation away from screens. If you want to develop your nervous system, you must give your body enough time to completely relax. You may unwind by taking a warm bath, breathing deeply in between meetings with clients, or just lounging and giving yourself a moment. Put your phone aside and give yourself some time to relax and clear your mind.

11. Proprioceptive stimulation

The body's capacity to sense its location in space while it moves is known as proprioception. Weight-bearing exercises (pushing, crawling), resistance exercises (pulling, pushing), heaving lifting, cardiovascular exercises (running, jumping), oral exercises (chewing), and deep pressure exercises (hugs!) can all be used to activate it. Your nervous system is supported and balanced when you engage in proprioceptive activities. Even if they don't take a lot of time or effort, some of them can still be beneficial forms of physical activity.

12. Cold plunges

Water with varying temperatures is necessary to restore equilibrium to an unbalanced neurological system. The many health advantages that cold treatment provides are the main reason for its significant rise in popularity in recent years. It has been demonstrated to help with anxiety, depression, and other mood disorders as well as nervous system regulation. Additionally, it frequently enhances immunological responses and quickens metabolism.

13. Meditation

Numerous benefits of meditation exist for stress, anxiety, melancholy, and sleeplessness. Additionally, it helps us better manage our thoughts and emotions by increasing our awareness of them. Studies reveal that meditation can modify the structure of the brain or even increase neuronal connections. You can select the kind of meditation that is best for you from a variety of options, including Zen meditation and mindfulness meditation. Your nervous system's health can be greatly impacted by taking even five deliberate breaths throughout the day!

14. Tech-free moments

Technology is becoming more and more important in our daily lives. We seem to never be able to go a minute without being plugged in, whether it is for our laptops or smartphones. One of the most overstimulating habits we all have is staring at our phone screens all day. Before you know it, you've wasted hours scrolling through Instagram and are feeling dysregulated due to a notice here and a message there. It develops into a powerful habit or perhaps an addiction that is difficult to break. In addition to its psychological effects, phone addiction has physical side effects. Some of the adverse consequences include melatonin suppression-related sleep disturbances and eye issues. For this reason, it's crucial to set aside some time each day without using electronics, especially in the evening before bed.

15. Sunshine

For good health, we need sunshine. Vitamin D, which is aided by sunlight, can help stabilize an unbalanced neurological system. The ideal time to enjoy the sun is early in the morning before it reaches its maximum UV value. A few more foods high in vitamin D include milk, eggs, and salmon. In addition, exposure to the sun raises serotonin levels, which control our mood. Going for a stroll in the sunshine seems like a beneficial thing we can do for our wellbeing, doesn't it? Just don't forget to use SPF cream to protect your skin.

16. Bathing in the outdoors or the forest

Spending time in nature has a special ability to relax and rejuvenate one. Perhaps it's the sight of towering trees above you or the sound of leaves rustling in the breeze. Whatever the cause, there's little doubt that spending time in nature can lower stress and increase well-being. Research has shown that spending time in nature can have positive effects on blood pressure, heart rate, and relaxation. A short stroll in a forest has been demonstrated to significantly lower stress markers. There are fewer pressures in the forest, allowing us to focus entirely on the peaceful sounds of the natural world.

17. Keep a journal to let go of old trauma

One excellent method to declutter is to put your negative ideas, traumatic experiences, and grievances in writing. This technique, which helps you reset your thinking, is frequently referred to as "mind dumping." Additionally, it may facilitate the management of challenging emotions that we may encounter for whatever reason. Writing is sometimes used as a therapeutic technique that has a therapeutic effect.

18. Baths with Epsom salts

Magnesium, which is present in Epsom salt baths, might improve mood by raising serotonin levels, which lowers stress. Epsom salts can help with muscle and nerve dysfunction. How about a scented candle and a soothing playlist while taking an Epsom salt bath? Just fill a warm bath with two cups of salt and soak for twenty minutes. That's something your nervous system will appreciate!

19. Somatic perception

A body-orienting method called somatic experiencing is intended to release tension that has become trapped in the body as a result of trauma or other abruptly traumatic prior events. By teaching people how to re-establish a connection with their bodies, somatic experiencing seeks to assist individuals manage their nervous system. Specific motions, soft touch, and mindfulness exercises can help achieve this. Through therapy work with body sensations, an educated practitioner guides the client toward safety and the development of self-regulation skills.

20. Exercises to relax the vagus nerve

The parasympathetic nervous system is triggered by the vagus nerve. It is related to the muscles in the back of your throat and your vocal cords. The vagus nerve can be physically stimulated by laughing, om-ing, singing, and gargling. Your vocal cords' tactile sensation can trigger the vagus nerve! Sing om-mantras, hum, laugh, chant, or do whatever else that comes naturally to you to help your nervous system.

21. The use of hypnosis

A hypnotherapist can assist you in achieving guided hypnosis through hypnotherapy. To assist patients in achieving a deep state of relaxation, it makes use of suggestion and guided relaxation. When the nervous system is in this state, it is more open to the therapist's constructive ideas. This can help with a variety of problems, such as worry, stress, pain management, and more. This trance-like experience is similar to losing yourself in a book, movie, or piece of music. It's capable of rewiring the brain.

22. Family structures within families

Certain "parts" of your personality can be managed with the aid of internal family systems. This method is based on the notion that each of us is the culmination of our various subpersonalities. It indicates that there is more to us than meets the eye of a single personality type. It's acceptable to feel lazy even when you put in a lot of work! Some of our subpersonalities, which can hinder us in our adult lives, are products of challenging childhood events. For instance, if you were traumatically injured as a youngster, you might have created a defense mechanism to keep yourself safe. Internal family processes can be helpful if you've been in this position for too long and need assistance leaving.

23. Tools for vibration and touch treatment

Touch and vibration treatment is offered by a variety of equipment offers touch and vibration treatments. When you experience an emotional state, they assist in teaching you how to change it. Some of these devices, like the Apollo, offer touch therapy, which merely vibrates your nervous system in a calming, silent manner to relax it. These vibrations inform your nervous system that you are in a safe location, allowing it to enter the resting and digesting state.

24. Heart rate variability (HRV) is on the rise

The time interval between heartbeats is measured by heart rate variability. It serves as a reliable gauge of the health of your neural system. You can enter a hyper-focused flow state and gain greater control over your subconscious feedback by using a variety of techniques that assess heart rate variability (HRV). How can you put it to use? Monitoring your heart rate variability (HRV) can help you avoid overtraining, avoid burnout from stress, and make health-related decisions. These devices are useful for monitoring everything from calories to heart rate variability!

25. Neurofeedback

A brand-new area of research called neurofeedback has emerged as a result of recent technological developments. This method of training and evaluating the nervous system is non-invasive. During the process, brainwaves are measured, and the patient receives immediate feedback regarding their brain's state.

Rebuilding circuits and increasing neural connectivity that foster safety and a sense of centering, may benefit people with dysregulated brains. Neurofeedback is frequently used in the treatment of attention-deficit/hyperactivity disorder. It focuses on using electroencephalogram (EEG) machines to alter how the brain reacts to various inputs.

26. Eye movements are desensitized and reprocessed

With EMDR, an eight-phase psychotherapy procedure, people can recover from emotional pain in their lives with the use of EMDR, an eight-phase psychotherapy procedure. To end emotional dysregulation, EMDR assists in retrieving traumatic memories and forming new, adaptive memories. What exactly is the operation mechanism? Following the first preparation, the patient attends to emotionally challenging feelings while focusing on outside stimuli, like lateral eye movements guided by the therapist.

27. Omega Three

The nervous system is in charge of transmitting messages throughout the body, and omega-3 fatty acids are necessary for the nervous system to function properly. These fats help with nerve cell insulation and damage prevention. Omega-3 fatty acids are abundant in DHA and EPA, which are essential for the development of the neurological system. They help maintain healthy neuron activity and enhance nerve transmission.

The majority of them are found in nuts and seeds (including flaxseed, chia seeds, and walnuts), fish and seafood (particularly cold-water fat fish), and plant oils (like soybean and flaxseed oil). Don't forget to include some of those in your regular diet!

28. Magnesium

One of the minerals that is necessary for a healthy neurological system is magnesium. Magnesium stimulates a relaxing response. A magnesium deficiency may impede multiple neurotransmitters that facilitate nerve signal transmission. This can lead to recurrent headaches, fatigue, insomnia, cramping in the legs, increased irritability, or shaking hands and eyes.

Consume a daily serving of buckwheat groats, almonds, oatmeal, pumpkin seeds, peas, or chickpeas to give your body the proper quantity of magnesium. You might also think about taking supplements. For magnesium to be efficiently absorbed, vitamin 6 is also required.

29. GABA

The body naturally produces the amino acid GABA. The brain's inhibitory neurotransmitter, GABA, is sometimes referred to as "the natural Valium" since it promotes greater cognitive function and a calmer mood. It improves focus, lessens the negative effects of stress, reduces levels of fear and anxiety, and may even aid with sleep issues. Low GABA levels can result in a tense or anxious feeling. This may make it challenging to focus or fall asleep.

Certain fermented foods, like kefir, sauerkraut, pickled beets or cucumbers, beetroot sourdough, and natural yogurt, contain GABA.

30. B complex vitamins

B vitamins are necessary nutrients that are involved in a wide range of bodily processes. The most significant benefit of B vitamins may be that they support healthy nervous system function. They help to synthesize neurotransmitters, which are involved in intercellular communication. If the body is lacking in B vitamins, the neurological system may be impacted, leading to numbness or pins and needles. In particular, B-12 is necessary to safeguard the coverings around nerves.

Nuts and seeds, beans, eggs, dairy products, chicken, bananas, peaches, and spinach are among the greatest foods to eat while looking for vitamin B vitamins. There is a wide range of vitamin B supplements available but always talk to your primary care physician before taking any.

31. L Theanine

Naturally present in tea leaves, the amino acid L-theanine enhances cognitive performance while also promoting relaxation.

Green tea and matcha contain L-theanine. If you have trouble sleeping, L-theanine may be able to help. It lowers levels of fear and anxiety and raises levels of serotonin, dopamine, and GABA, which are linked to happiness. It facilitates mental deceleration, relaxation, and falling asleep.

32. John's Wort

Popular herbal treatment St. John's Wort has been used for millennia to cure a wide range of ailments. These days, its most well-known use is in treating anxiety and depressive symptoms. St. John's Wort is a nervous system tonic and brain adaptogen. It can be used therapeutically, strengthening and revitalizing the neurological system. You can apply this plant physically or orally. It is used to treat mild to moderate depression because of its therapeutic effects.

33. Electrolytes

Your nervous system is in charge of sending messages throughout your body, and for it to work correctly, electrolytes are necessary. Without the right ratios of sodium, potassium, magnesium, and calcium, nerves cannot operate normally. These electrolytes allow for adequate neuronal signaling, cardiac contractions, and muscular contractions. In particular, coconut water is a great provider of electrolytes. Don't worry if you don't live in an area where coconut palms tower above you! Coconut water is sold worldwide and exported extensively.

34. Blood sugar equilibrium

For general health and well-being, it is imperative to maintain a healthy blood sugar balance. Excessive or insufficient blood sugar levels can significantly affect the neurological system. After a blood sugar increase, depression, worry, and exhaustion follow. Maintaining blood sugar homeostasis through self-monitoring is critical for mood control and dysregulation support. Devices for monitoring blood sugar levels can help achieve this.

Blood sugar surges can be avoided by following a low-carb and low-sugar diet, preserving a healthy weight, and engaging in regular exercise and hydration.

35. Fasting

The body can benefit from stress! For millennia, people have employed fasting as a means of fostering both spiritual and physical well-being. The body can relax and repair itself when there is a temporary fast from food and liquids. Fasting has the potential to effectively balance an unbalanced neurological system and enhance concentration and mental clarity. Hormesis, a kind of stress, encourages the body to adapt and grow more resilient. According to certain research, fasting can dramatically quiet your sympathetic nervous system and activate your parasympathetic nervous system, which indicates that your fight or flight response will be suppressed and your rest and digest mode will be activated.

36. Superior nutrition, staying away from processed foods, and consuming a lot of fermented foods

For the nervous system to develop and operate properly, nutrition is necessary. The neurological system needs a lot of minerals and vitamins. As a result, it is critical to consume complete, unprocessed meals. Healthy fats also serve the purpose of insulation. There is also research on eating fermented foods for a happier gut. Look at the quality of the items you purchase to make sure they can support your health the next time you go grocery shopping. Numerous applications are available to assist you in this regard; all you have to do is scan the product barcodes to obtain comprehensive details regarding their composition and caliber.

37. Caffeine & Yerba Mate

Caffeine is one tool that can be used. It has stimulating properties that aid in keeping people awake and focused. According to studies, yerba mate can increase energy, promote mental clarity, and possibly aid in illness prevention. Small doses can have positive effects like increased energy and attention, but large doses can cause anxiety and agitate us by triggering our fight-or-flight response. To prevent coffee and other stimulating beverages from impairing your sleep, try to avoid drinking them in the evening.

38. Limit your intake of alcohol

The human body is susceptible to several short- and long-term impacts from alcohol intake. When taken in excess, it can cause vomiting, coma, and even death. In the short term, it can impair cognitive function and motor skills. Alcohol damages the central nervous system by interfering with proper communication between brain receptors. Drinking alcohol for an extended period can harm the neurological system, resulting in balance issues, sluggish reaction times, disorientation, and diminished attentiveness.

While there may be some health benefits associated with moderate drinking, the hazards associated with excessive drinking much outweigh any potential advantages. Alcohol can be a healthy lifestyle component when used moderately; when misused, though, it can wreck lives.

39. Adaptogens

a. Ashwagandha

Indian ashwagandha has been used for ages to treat a wide range of ailments. This herb has therapeutic properties that help reduce tension and anxiety, strengthening the neurological system as a result. Because it is an adaptogen, it assists the body in adjusting to stimuli. According to research, it may help alleviate anxiety and insomnia, enhance cognitive abilities, and lower blood sugar. Ashwagandha is now offered in many different forms, including tinctures, powders, and capsules.

b. Rhodiola

Traditional medical systems have utilized the plant Rhodiola rosea. It grows in the chilly parts of Asia and Europe. These days, a plethora of health advantages are recognized in it, one of which is the nervous system's support. Research indicates that it could aid in the regulation of emotions, mood, and anxiety by reducing the activity of the sympathetic nervous system. Apart from its advantageous effects on the neurological system, Rhodiola is also recognized for elevating energy levels, improving cognitive abilities, and decreasing inflammation.

c. Ginseng

For millennia, people have utilized ginseng for its therapeutic benefits. It is believed that ginseng's active components are good for the nervous system. This plant has adaptogenic properties that aid the body in adjusting to both physical and mental strain. Among its many advantages are its ability to cure chronic fatigue syndrome, anxiety, and depression. Its antioxidant content might lessen inflammation. It is advisable to see a healthcare provider before taking ginseng to be sure it is appropriate for you.

40. Plants (Oat straw)

Because it is a nervine plant, oat straw extract is a "hug for your nervous system," helping to restore a dysregulated neurological system. B vitamins, which are abundant in oat straw, can help with fatigue, anxiety, sadness, and issues with memory and attention. It might also enhance blood flow and lessen inflammation. Oat straw is useful in a variety of forms, such as tea and capsules, but it works best as an extract or tincture. These concentrated versions benefit the nervous system the most and facilitate the body's easier absorption of nutrients in oat straw.

41. Teas

a. Tea with chamomile

Chamomile is used to ease anxiety and soothe tense muscles. Research indicates that chamomile enhances the functioning of the central nervous system by altering the brain's alpha-wave activity, which facilitates relaxation. It is often used as a home treatment for indigestion and upset stomachs.

Apart from its relaxing properties, chamomile tea contains antioxidants that can strengthen the immune system and shield cells from harm. Are you having trouble sleeping? For that, you might try having a cup of chamomile tea!

b. Matcha with green tea

L-theanine, an ingredient in green tea, can raise serotonin and dopamine levels. These have a beneficial impact on stress and mood. Antioxidants included in green tea can strengthen the autonomic nervous system and improve attention, alertness, and attentiveness. When compared to coffee or other caffeinated beverages, matcha is often found to offer a more balanced energy boost. Try substituting green tea or matcha for coffee if you want to cut back on your regular intake and gain some additional energy from them.

42. Setting boundaries

When you establish boundaries, you take care of your needs and protect yourself. They are also essential for establishing wholesome interpersonal relationships. You will probably feel overwhelmed and have less energy than normal if individuals are consistently stepping over your limits. When your energy level is low, you could find it difficult to control your emotions. Setting limits is a crucial part of effective management.

43. The use of acupuncture

Acupuncture is one type of traditional Chinese medicine that has been used for generations. The fundamental idea of acupuncture is that the body is made up of energy lines, and blockages in these lines can result in disease or discomfort. To restore balance and health, tiny needles are inserted into certain spots along these energy channels. Acupuncture opens the body's meridians to increase blood flow and energy, which can reset the nervous system. It can encourage relaxation, which triggers a parasympathetic state. It might also help you with some medical conditions including migrens, spinal disorders, or degenerative joint diseases, depending on the situation.

44. Build healthy relationships

One of the most healing practices is being in healthy relationships where we feel free to be who we are! They have been demonstrated to affect recovery, stress management, and general health. Having a real buddy we can confide in during trying times is invaluable and aids in emotional self-control. Research indicates that preserving a positive, healthy relationship may potentially extend one's life!

45. Heal your attachment style

Childhood experiences shape one's attachment style, which persists throughout adulthood. It's based on our early interactions with caretakers and how they respond to our demands. When our wants are consistently and tenderly met, we form a secure connection pattern. We become attached in an insecure manner if our wants are not regularly addressed or if we are neglected, we become insecurely attached. Our ability to operate in relationships as adults is significantly impacted by attachment trauma experienced as children. For instance, if our father abandoned us, we can have ongoing anxiety because we think our spouse will follow suit. might you observe any such tendencies in your life, you might think about addressing them in therapy.

Signs of a Well-Regulated Neurological System and their Significance

The following are some indicators of a well-regulated nervous system, as well as the reasons why they are important for your overall health:

- The capacity for clear thought. A well-balanced neurological system enables us to think clearly and express ourselves more efficiently because it prevents mental fog.

- You feel confident in yourself.

- Always present in the moment and able to engage in lively dialogue and conversations

- Extremely willing to have fun. Having a controlled nervous system allows one to be carefree, wacky, and humorous.

- We avoid overanalyzing circumstances and can think rationally without going overboard

- The heart rate is constant.

- We breathe in a manner that calms our bodies by doing so slowly.

Scientific treatments for nervous system dysregulation

For a very long time, scientists have been studying and researching the dysregulated neural system to help victims reset their nervous systems and reduce stress hormones. Scientists have provided numerous responses and determined what is effective and ineffective.

Two scientific treatments were developed to assist in resetting the dysregulated neurological system:

1. Band-Aid solution for controlling the nervous system (ineffective)
2. The limbic system malfunctions (works).

A temporary solution for nervous system control

The mechanical engineers offered this as a long-term scientific answer to help regulate the neurological system. It was designed to detect and monitor patients' muscle activity before medication, and it is the size of a plaster. Sadly, it didn't work for the reasons listed below:

- Insufficient storage capacity as a result of several onboard electronics

- Inexplicable energy consumption

- There was no suitable method for delivering medication via the skin.

- The device's electrical parts weren't made to be in contact with human skin.

- The limb system is dysfunctional.

The brain networking system, which has been successful in controlling the neurological system, is also in charge of shaping people's memories and emotions.

The limbic cortex, hippocampus formation, septal area, hypothalamus, and amygdala make up the system. From a biological standpoint, these structures have effectively collaborated with other brain regions to govern physiological and psychological processes like as memory, emotions, and even sexual desire, ultimately aiding in nervous system regulation.

Six steps to nervous system regulation

1. **Deep inhaling**

   Basic practices, like as inhaling deeply, are vital and assist in nervous system regulation. By activating the parasympathetic nervous system and bringing the body back to a relaxed, peaceful state, deep breathing exercises help the body recognize that everything is okay at this point.

   Box breathing exercises are suggested by several scientists and doctors. These exercises consist of four simple stages that match the four sides of a box. To feel the air entering your lungs, first take a deep breath and slowly count to four. Secondly, try not to breathe in or out during the four seconds you hold your breath. After that, you can take a four-second, gentle breath out through your mouth. Just repeat steps one through three until you feel re-centered, which is the last step.

2. **Let your shoulders and neck drop**

   People frequently feel tension in the neck and shoulders due to stress and anxiety. If not treated or cured, chronic pain and other health problems may result from this if it is not treated or cured. But fear not—yoga, stretching, and other stress-reduction techniques can help relieve muscle tightness in the shoulders and neck.

3. **Spreading a smile across your face**

You can trick your brain into thinking you're happy just by smiling. Whether forced or real, smiling can alter your mood and elevate your mental condition, according to two studies done in Wales and Germany. A simple smile can help you recover from the negative consequences of unresolved tension and maintain your composure.

4. **Take brisk walks outside or morning and evening runs**

Running and walking are two activities that promote calmness and relaxation. The nervous system can also be regulated by various exercises such as weightlifting, yoga, aerobics, and stretching.

5. **Hug a love one**

   Although it may sound cliched and outdated, cuddling has been shown to promote calmness in people. Oxytocin, the hormone associated with love, is known to help people relax and cope with stress.

6. **Strive to think more positively and steer clear of negative thoughts**

   Negative thoughts can overtake a person due to a dysregulated neurological system, claims Dr. Leaf. Nonetheless, this may be effectively managed by ensuring that you focus on three or four constructive ideas and keep yourself from giving in to pessimistic thinking.

   These optimistic ideas might be built upon your best-loved ones—books, movies, music, joyful recollections, enthusiastic plans for the future, or even a truly amazing moment of making love.

Summing Up

This chapter provides techniques for restoring a dysregulated neurological system, which can lead to anxiety, burnout, and trauma. These techniques can help raise energy levels, reduce stress and anxiety, improve sleep quality, and promote overall health and well-being.

There is no universal solution for treating a dysregulated nervous system, but some basic recommendations include lifestyle modifications like better eating, consistent exercise, and good sleep hygiene. Body-mind exercises like yoga, meditation, or breathwork may be helpful for others, while therapists and supplements may be beneficial for those with high sensitivity.

Some techniques work best for individuals with a dysregulated nervous system, such as 7-9 hours of undisturbed, deep sleep, deep inhalation, moderate exercise, co-regulation in a safe relationship with a loved one, Qi Gong, Tai Chi, and yoga. These ancient techniques help develop bodily balance and relaxation, lower stress, and enhance general wellness.

Chanting and singing are also powerful methods for calming the nervous system. Chanting involves repeatedly using the same word or phrase, aiding in mental clarity and attention. Singing triggers the vagus nerve and slows respiration, making vocal stimulation a quick route from fight-or-flight to rest and digestion.

In conclusion, the text emphasizes the importance of various techniques for restoring a dysregulated neurological system, including deep sleep, deep breathing, moderate exercise, co-regulation in a safe relationship, yoga, chanting, and meditation. By implementing these strategies, individuals can improve their overall well-being and overall well-being.

Go barefoot on unpaved surfaces, massages, aromas, and unstructured downtime can help calm the nervous system and reduce stress. Nature's calming effects on the human mind have been scientifically proven to aid in stress reduction, inflammation, heart rate variability, improved sleep, cortisol management, and autonomic nervous system balance. Massage therapy stimulates the parasympathetic division, promoting better sleep and focus.

Aromas can also reduce stress by eliciting feelings and memories, while scents can lower brain stress signals. Unstructured downtime and leisure away from screens are crucial for developing the nervous system. Engaging in proprioception exercises, such as weight-bearing, resistance, and cardiovascular exercises, can support and balance the nervous system. Cold descents with varying temperatures can restore equilibrium and improve mood disorders, immunological responses, and metabolism.

Meditation has numerous benefits for stress, anxiety, melancholy, sleeplessness, and better management of thoughts and emotions. Studies show that meditation can modify the structure of the brain or increase neuronal connections. Tech-free moments, such as avoiding phone screens, are essential for maintaining good health. Sunlight, particularly early in the morning, can help stabilize an unbalanced neurological system and raise serotonin levels, which control mood.

Bathing in nature or the outdoors can also relax and rejuvenate the body. Spending time in nature can lower stress and increase well-being by reducing blood pressure, heart rate, and relaxation.

The text provides a list of techniques and tools to help individuals manage their trauma and emotional states. Some of these techniques include keeping a journal, baths with Epsom salts, somatic perception, hypnosis, family structures within families, touch and vibration treatment, heart rate variability (HRV), neurofeedback, eye movements desensitization and reprocessing, omega-3 fatty acids, and incorporating them into one's diet.

Writing is an effective method for decluttering and managing negative thoughts and experiences. Epsom salt baths can improve mood by raising serotonin levels, lowering stress, and helping with muscle and nerve dysfunction. Somatic perception involves releasing tension trapped in the body due to trauma or other traumatic events. Exercises to relax the vagus nerve, which is related to the muscles in the back of the throat and vocal cords, can help manage the nervous system.

Hypnosis can help individuals achieve guided relaxation and manage various problems such as worry, stress, and pain management. Internal family systems can help manage certain aspects of one's personality, such as subpersonalities formed from challenging childhood events. Touch and vibration treatment can help manage emotional states by vibrating the nervous system in a calming, silent manner.

Neurofeedback is a non-invasive method of training and evaluating the nervous system, focusing on building circuits and increasing neural connectivity. Eye movements are desensitized and reprocessed through EMDR, an eight-phase psychotherapy procedure that helps people recover from emotional pain. Omega-3 fatty acids, such as DHA and EPA, are essential for the development of the neurological system and help maintain healthy neuron activity and enhance nerve transmission.

Magnesium is essential for a healthy neurological system, as it stimulates a relaxing response and can prevent neurotransmitter deficiencies. Consuming buckwheat groats, almonds, oatmeal, pumpkin seeds, peas, or chickpeas can provide magnesium, while taking supplements is also recommended. GABA, the brain's inhibitory neurotransmitter, promotes cognitive function and a calmer mood. Consuming fermented foods like kefir, sauerkraut, pickled beets, cucumbers, beetroot sourdough, and natural yogurt contains GABA. B complex vitamins, such as B-12, support healthy nervous system function and help synthesize neurotransmitters involved in intercellular communication.

Theanine L, found in tea leaves, enhances cognitive performance and promotes relaxation. Green tea and matcha contain L-theanine, which can help with sleep issues by lowering fear and anxiety and increasing serotonin, dopamine, and GABA levels. St. John's Wort, a nervous system tonic and brain adaptogen, can be used to treat anxiety and depressive symptoms.

Electrolytes are necessary for the nervous system to function properly. Maintaining a healthy blood sugar balance is crucial for mood control and dysregulation support. Self-monitoring blood sugar levels can help achieve this. A low-carb and low-sugar diet, maintaining a healthy weight, and regular exercise and hydration can help prevent blood sugar surges.

Fasting has been used for centuries to foster spiritual and physical well-being, and fasting can help balance an unbalanced neurological system. Consuming complete, unprocessed meals, healthy fats, and fermented foods can support the nervous system. Coffee and Mate Herbal Tea can also be beneficial, with small doses increasing energy and attention but large doses potentially causing anxiety and agitation.

Alcohol consumption can have both short- and long-term effects on the human body, including damage to the central nervous system and impaired cognitive function. Moderate drinking can be beneficial, but excessive drinking can lead to severe health issues.

Adaptogens like ashwagandha, Rhodiola, and ginseng can help reduce tension, anxiety, and strengthen the nervous system. Ashwagandha is known for its therapeutic properties, while Rhodiola supports the nervous system by reducing sympathetic nervous system activity. Ginseng, on the other hand, has adaptogenic properties that help the body adjust to physical and mental strain.

Oat straw extract is a nervine plant that can help restore a dysregulated neurological system by enhancing blood flow and reducing inflammation. Teas like tea with chamomile and matcha with green tea can also help with stress and mood by raising serotonin and dopamine levels.

Establishing limits is crucial for effective management and maintaining healthy interpersonal relationships. Acupuncture, a traditional Chinese medicine, uses needles to restore balance and health by opening the body's meridians, promoting relaxation and potentially treating medical conditions like migraines, spinal disorders, and degenerative joint diseases.

Creating healthy connections is another important practice for healing, as they can affect recovery, stress management, and overall health. Maintaining positive, healthy relationships can potentially extend one's life.

Attachment styles, shaped by childhood experiences, significantly impact adult relationships. A well-regulated neurological system is crucial for overall health, allowing clear thought, confidence, active engagement, and enjoyment. Scientists have developed treatments to reset the nervous system and reduce stress hormones. Two treatments are Band-Aid and the limbic system malfunctions.

The Band-Aid was designed to monitor muscle activity before medication but failed due to insufficient storage capacity, energy consumption, and incompatible electrical parts. The limbic system, consisting of the limbic cortex, hippocampus formation, septal area, hypothalamus, and amygdala, has been successful in controlling the neurological system.

Six steps to nervous system regulation include deep inhaling, letting your shoulders and neck drop, spreading a smile across your face, taking brisk walks, hugging a loved one, and striving to think more positively. Deep breathing exercises activate the parasympathetic nervous system, while box breathing exercises help relax muscles. Spreading a smile can trick the brain into thinking you're happy, while running and walking promote calmness and relaxation. Hugging a loved one can also help relax and cope with stress.

To restore a healthy attachment style, it's essential to focus on positive thoughts and avoid pessimistic thinking. Building on positive experiences like books, movies, music, or romantic moments can help manage negative thoughts and improve overall well-being.

www.ingramcontent.com/pod-product-compliance
Lightning Source LLC
Chambersburg PA
CBHW071040250726
48653CB00005B/1926